DEFEATING LUPUS WITH EXPERT GUIDANCE

Ultimate Solution Handbook For Patients, Guardians Or Family To Understand, Manage, Treat, Prevent, Reverse Symptoms And Live Well

DR. POTTER WHITLEY

Copyright © 2023 by Dr. Potter Whitley

DISCLAIMER:

This book's contents are meant to be used solely for informative purposes. The information should not be used as a replacement for expert medical advice, diagnosis, or care.

The information contained in this book is accurate and reliable, having been verified by the author to the best of his ability. Nevertheless, the author disclaims all express and implied representations and warranties regarding the availability, correctness, appropriateness, completeness, and reliability of the material provided here. You bear full responsibility for any reliance you may have on such material.

For informational purposes, this book may make reference to or mention of certain people, things, websites, organizations, or other names. The author has no connection to, endorsement from, or recommendation for these organizations. The author's approval or validation is not implied by the inclusion of these references.

Any direct, indirect, incidental, special, or consequential damages resulting from using or not being able to use the material in this book are not covered by the author's liability policy. For medical advice and counsel particular to their circumstances, readers are advised to check with experienced healthcare specialists.

The content, materials, and information in this book are subject to change at any time without prior notice, at the author's discretion. The text may contain errors or omissions for which the author is not responsible.

By reading this book, you understand and accept the conditions of this disclaimer.

THE REASON BEHIND THIS BOOK

"Defeating Lupus With Expert Guidance" proves to be an invaluable tool for people attempting to navigate the intricacies of lupus, providing a thorough examination that delves deeper than the surface knowledge of this inflammatory disease. The first few chapters cover the basics, explaining the mystery of lupus by concentrating on its various manifestations, underlying causes, and possible triggers. This background information gives readers a strong platform on which to understand the complex ways that lupus presents itself in the body.

The importance of this work is increased even more as it delves into the complex area of the effect on the body. Through analyzing immune system failure and pinpointing the organs at risk for lupus, readers can comprehend the complex network of symptoms and flare-ups that define this illness. Interestingly, the focus on early diagnosis in later chapters is a proactive strategy that highlights how important it is to identify symptoms and get tested to improve treatment results.

This book's approach to treating lupus is one of its strong points. It explores lifestyle modifications that are crucial for treating lupus in addition to outlining drugs and their particular functions. Complementary therapies are included because they recognize the complexity of managing lupus and provide a holistic approach. Most importantly, this book is unique in that it presents professional opinions and highlights the joint efforts of lupus experts and rheumatologists. Building a strong healthcare team is facilitated for readers, with a focus on the team approach required for successful treatment.

This book's emphasis on trigger detection, emergency preparedness, and coping mechanisms makes navigating the turbulent waters of lupus flares more bearable. With empathy, the relationship between lupus and mental health is examined, recognizing the emotional toll and providing coping strategies. This book also acknowledges the critical role that nutrition plays in managing lupus, outlining an anti-inflammatory diet and how supplements affect symptoms.

The holistic requirements of people with lupus are acknowledged, and lifestyle modifications, stress management, and the development of a supportive network are given the attention they deserve. This book also discusses the special difficulties that lupus presents during pregnancy, offering priceless advice on preparation, dangers, and postpartum issues.

This book, an enlightening beacon, doesn't hide from the future; in fact, a portion is devoted to research and the changing face of lupus treatment. It clarifies recent findings, newly developed treatments, and the critical role that activism plays in raising public knowledge of lupus. "Defeating Lupus With Expert Guidance" is all things considered, more than just an instructional manual; it is a kind companion on the path to comprehending, controlling, and overcoming lupus.

TABLE OF CONTENT

CHAPTER ONE

INTRODUCTION TO LUPUS
What is lupus?

Systemic lupus erythematosus (SLE), the formal name for lupus, is a chronic, multifaceted autoimmune illness that can impact many body parts. The immune system, which is meant to defend the body against dangerous intruders like bacteria and viruses, attacks its tissues and organs when a person has lupus. This leads to pain, inflammation, and harm to the kidneys, heart, lungs, blood vessels, joints, skin, and brain. Although the precise etiology of lupus is unknown, a mix of hormonal, environmental, and genetic variables are thought to be involved.

The unpredictability of lupus is one of its distinguishing characteristics. The severity of the symptoms might vary, and they frequently flare up and disappear at different times. Fever, rashes on the skin, joint pain, and exhaustion are typical symptoms.

But lupus is dubbed the "great imitator" because it can be difficult to identify. After all, its symptoms might resemble those of a variety of other conditions. This frequently results in cases being delayed or misdiagnosed, which makes managing the illness more difficult.

Managing lupus necessitates continuous medical attention, and the standard course of treatment entails a mix of drugs to manage symptoms and avoid exacerbations. Moreover, alterations in lifestyle, like stress reduction, consistent exercise, and sun protection, are vital for the successful management of lupus.

Lupus Types

There are various types of lupus, and each has unique symptoms and effects on the body. Systemic lupus erythematosus (SLE) is the most prevalent type and affects many organs and systems in the body. The skin is the main organ affected by cutaneous lupus erythematosus, leading to lesions and rashes.

Skin is the only organ affected by discoid lupus erythematosus, which frequently results in disk-shaped, circular lesions. Certain drugs have the potential to cause drug-induced lupus, which often goes away when the prescription is stopped.

It is significant to remember that lupus is a highly individualized disease, with substantial individual variation in its presentation. While skin or organ involvement may be experienced by some, joint and muscle pain may be the main complaint for others. The variety of lupus forms complicates diagnosis and therapy, necessitating a customized strategy based on the particular needs and symptoms of each patient.

Reasons and Initiators

Although the precise causes of lupus are still unknown, a mix of hormonal, environmental, and genetic variables are thought to have a role in the disease's development. A genetic predisposition is involved, as lupus is more common in people with a family history of autoimmune illnesses.

Environmental factors can potentially hasten the onset of lupus, especially in those who are genetically predisposed. These factors include exposure to specific infections, sunshine, and drugs.

Given that women of reproductive age are disproportionately affected by lupus, hormonal factors, notably the action of estrogen, are assumed to have a role in the disease. Hormone fluctuations, including those brought on by pregnancy or the use of oral contraceptives, might affect how a disease manifests itself.

One of the most important parts of managing lupus is recognizing and controlling triggers. Preventing flare-ups requires careful monitoring of medications, minimizing stress, and avoiding excessive sun exposure. Regular medical check-ups also facilitate early diagnosis of potential issues and enable treatment plans to be modified.

In conclusion, it is critical for medical professionals and those who are afflicted with lupus to comprehend the complex interactions of genetic, environmental, and hormonal components in the development of the disease. Effective management and enhancing the quality of life for lupus patients require a comprehensive strategy that takes into account the particulars of each patient's experience.

CHAPTER TWO

EFFECTS ON THE HUMAN BODY
Immune System Impairment:

A long-term autoimmune condition called lupus mostly affects the immune system, making it malfunction and target healthy tissues. The immune system's purpose is to protect the body from pathogens and other outside invaders like viruses. But in those who have lupus, the body's tissues and cells are misinterpreted by the immune system as enemies, which sets off a series of inflammatory reactions. The synthesis of autoantibodies, or antibodies that target and harm normal cells, is a sign of immune system malfunction.

One of the main causes of immunological dysfunction associated with lupus is the dysregulation of T and B cells, which are vital immune system constituents. T cells, which control the immune system, become hyperactive and cause tissue damage and inflammation. On the other side, B cells overproduce autoantibodies, which intensifies the assault on healthy cells. An ongoing state of inflammation is caused by a disruption in the complex balance of the immune system, which can affect many organs and systems in the body.

It is essential to comprehend the complexities of immune system failure in lupus to create appropriate treatment plans. To reestablish equilibrium without endangering immune system performance as a whole, researchers are investigating tailored medicines to modify particular immune pathways. Through the process of dissecting immunological dysregulation in lupus, professionals can customize interventions aimed at addressing the underlying causes of the illness and reducing the likelihood of flare-ups.

Organs Experiencing Lupus:

A multisystemic autoimmune disease, lupus can impact many different body tissues and organs. Lupus affects not just the skin and joints but also important organs like the heart, lungs, kidneys, and central nervous system. Because lupus nephritis, an inflammation of the kidneys, is a common consequence that, if left untreated, can cause substantial renal damage, the kidneys are especially sensitive.

Lupus can cause inflammation of the heart, and blood vessels, and possibly the onset of atherosclerosis as a cardiovascular symptom. This increased risk of cardiovascular complications highlights the systemic character of lupus and highlights the necessity of all-encompassing therapeutic strategies.

Pleuritis, or inflammation of the lining surrounding the lungs, is one way that pulmonary problems in lupus can present as chest pain and discomfort. Furthermore, lupus can affect the central nervous system, which can result in seizures, cognitive impairment, and in extreme situations, neuropsychiatric lupus.

Comprehending the wide range of organs impacted by lupus is vital in customizing therapy regimens that cater to individual patient requirements. To effectively address the complicated and variable signs of lupus, a multidisciplinary strategy combining rheumatologists, nephrologists, cardiologists, and other experts is often required.

Typical Signs and Feelings:

A wide range of symptoms, from moderate to severe, can be experienced with lupus, and these symptoms are frequently variable, with flare-ups—periods of elevated disease activity—present. Fatigue, photosensitivity, rashes on the skin (especially the recognizable butterfly rash on the face), joint discomfort, and swelling are common symptoms. Because of these frequent waxing and waning symptoms, lupus is a difficult condition to manage.

People may suffer a worsening of their symptoms during flares, along with heightened immune system activity and inflammation. Numerous things, including stress, infections, and UV radiation exposure, can cause these flare-ups. To effectively avoid and manage flare-ups, patients and healthcare professionals must have a thorough understanding of the triggers that cause flare-ups.

Furthermore, lupus is notorious for its unpredictable character, which makes it challenging to predict when symptoms may become better or worse. This unpredictability highlights how crucial it is for patients and their healthcare team to regularly assess and communicate so that treatment regimens can be modified as necessary. More specialized and focused methods for managing symptoms and preventing flare-ups are being made possible by developments in personalized medicine and the discovery of biomarkers linked to lupus activity.

CHAPTER THREE

IDENTIFICATION AND PROMPT RECOGNITION
Identifying Signs of Lupus:

The symptoms of lupus, a complicated inflammatory illness, can differ greatly from person to person. Early intervention and successful management depend on the ability to recognize these indicators. A characteristic sign is the appearance of a butterfly-shaped rash on the cheekbones and nose, which is commonly known as the malar rash. This particular skin symptom in addition to photosensitivity—the skin becoming abnormally sensitive to sunlight—may serve as a first indication of lupus.

One typical symptom that frequently mimics rheumatoid arthritis is joint pain and swelling. But lupus stands out because it affects many organ systems and results in symptoms including exhaustion, fever, and weight loss.

Severe symptoms like shortness of breath, renal malfunction, and chest pain can arise when internal organs are involved. A precise diagnosis requires an understanding of how these various symptoms interact with one another.

In addition, lupus is well known for its unpredictable course, which includes flare-ups and remissions. Because of its erratic nature, identification can be difficult, therefore it's important to be on the lookout for potential symptoms. To promote early diagnosis and efficient disease management, people should pay attention to persistent symptoms and swiftly visit healthcare specialists.

Diagnostic Procedures and Tests:

A combination of clinical assessment and specialized diagnostic testing is necessary for an accurate diagnosis of lupus. Blood testing is essential, and the main marker is antinuclear antibodies (ANA). Most cases of lupus have elevated ANA levels, which are indicative of an overworked immune system.

It is crucial to remember that additional testing is frequently necessary to diagnose lupus; a positive ANA test alone does not do so.

Anti-double-stranded DNA (anti-dsDNA) and anti-Smith antibodies, which are more specific to lupus, are two examples of particular antibodies that may be tested for in addition to other blood testing.

Additionally measured are complement levels, which are proteins involved in immunological responses. Imaging tests, like ultrasounds and X-rays, can be performed to determine the degree of organ involvement.

To establish conclusive proof of lupus, a biopsy of the afflicted tissues—such as the kidney or skin—may be advised in some circumstances. With the use of these diagnostic tools, medical experts can create individualized treatment regimens by gaining a thorough grasp of the disease's effects on the body.

The Significance of Prompt Awareness

Improving overall prognosis and avoiding irreparable organ damage need early lupus identification. Given that lupus is unpredictable and can impact important organs, prompt action is imperative. Targeted therapy approaches, such as immunosuppressive drugs, anti-inflammatory pharmaceuticals, and lifestyle changes, can be put into place with early detection.

Furthermore, prompt diagnosis enables lupus patients to take an active role in their medical treatment. It offers a chance to learn about coping mechanisms, lifestyle modifications, and symptom management. Healthcare providers can better control disease activity, reduce the risk of complications, and improve the quality of life for lupus patients by starting treatment early.

Beyond the advantages for the individual, early detection advances the knowledge and research on lupus. It advances the creation of more specialized and efficient treatments by enabling the identification of putative biomarkers and therapeutic targets. Essentially, early identification affects more than just the individual; it also has an impact on the larger field of lupus research, treatment, and advocacy.

CHAPTER FOUR

METHODS OF TREATING LUPUS
The Functions of Drugs in the Treatment of Lupus:

To effectively manage lupus, a combination of drugs designed to modulate the immune system and address particular symptoms is frequently necessary. Ibuprofen and other nonsteroidal anti-inflammatory medications (NSAIDs) are frequently used to treat lupus-related pain and inflammation. Although corticosteroids, like prednisone, are potent anti-inflammatory medications that can help control severe symptoms, prolonged use of these medications may have negative side effects.

Another family of pharmaceuticals used in the treatment of lupus is called disease-modifying antirheumatic drugs (DMARDs). A common DMARD administered to treat symptoms and stop flare-ups is hydroxychloroquine. Mycophenolate mofetil and azathioprine are examples of immunosuppressants that suppress the immune system to stop it from attacking healthy organs. Biologics are more recent medications that target particular immune system components to reduce inflammation associated with lupus, such as belimumab.

The severity of the illness, the patient's symptoms, and any possible side effects all influence the prescription selection. For best results, the drug schedule must be regularly reviewed and adjusted. To guarantee the most efficient and well-tolerated care, patients and their healthcare providers must have open communication.

Modifying Your Lifestyle to Manage Your Lupus:

Apart from pharmaceutical interventions, alterations in lifestyle are crucial for the management of lupus and enhancing general health. Getting enough sleep and controlling your stress levels are crucial elements of a lupus-friendly lifestyle. People with lupus often experience fatigue, so they need to prioritize getting enough sleep to aid in their body's repair and recuperation.

To keep muscles from atrophying and to maintain joint flexibility, regular exercise that is customized to each person's strengths and limits is essential. Finding a balance is crucial, though, since overdoing it can aggravate symptoms and cause weariness. Getting advice from medical specialists like physical therapists might help develop a customized fitness regimen.

Making dietary changes is crucial for managing lupus. An anti-inflammatory diet high in fruits, vegetables, and omega-3 fatty acids may be beneficial for certain lupus patients. Furthermore, as sunlight can cause or exacerbate lupus symptoms, limiting sun exposure and wearing sunscreen are essential.

An essential component of lupus management is emotional health. People who are suffering from a chronic illness can benefit from support groups, counseling, and mindfulness exercises. Building a solid network of friends and family to lean on can be very helpful in overcoming the challenges of living with lupus.

Alternative Medicines for Lupus:

Complementary treatments can be incorporated into the lupus treatment plan to improve quality of life and improve symptom control. These therapies can be beneficial supplements to traditional treatments, even if they are not a replacement for medical measures.

For instance, acupuncture has been investigated as a supplemental treatment for pain and exhaustion associated with lupus. Certain bodily locations can be gently stimulated to provide relief for some people. Another treatment that might ease tense muscles and encourage relaxation is massage therapy.

Mind-body practices, like yoga and meditation, are becoming more widely acknowledged for their possible advantages in the treatment of lupus symptoms. These techniques emphasize unwinding, lowering stress levels, and enhancing well-being.

Because of its soft motions, tai chi may also aid people with lupus by increasing their flexibility and balance.

Lupus patients must consult their healthcare provider about any alternative therapies to make sure they are safe and suitable for their particular circumstances. Although these therapies might provide some symptom alleviation, conventional medical treatments should still be used in conjunction with them, not in substitute for them. An integrated strategy that incorporates lifestyle modifications, complementary therapies, and medicine can offer a comprehensive approach to controlling lupus and enhancing overall quality of life.

CHAPTER FIVE

PROFESSIONAL PERSPECTIVES ON LUPUS TREATMENT
Specialists In Lupus And Rheumatology:

The crucial significance that rheumatologists and lupus specialists play in the complex field of lupus care cannot be emphasized. These healthcare providers provide specific knowledge and insights into the intricate dynamics of an autoimmune disease, making them the cornerstone of a patient's journey. Particularly skilled in the diagnosis and treatment of disorders affecting the joints, muscles, and bones, rheumatologists play a crucial role in the management of lupus, which frequently presents with symptoms affecting these regions.

On the other hand, lupus specialists have a detailed understanding of all the aspects of the disease, from its immunological foundations to the varied ways it can present in different people. Their specialist knowledge makes it possible to treat patients in a more focused and efficient manner, guaranteeing that they receive individualized care that caters to the unique details of their disease.

Building a solid and open line of communication with these experts is essential. Patients can talk about symptomatology, available treatments, and the overall impact of the disease on their quality of life at routine visits. Through active patient participation in healthcare decision-making, this collaborative approach cultivates a sense of shared responsibility.

Because lupus has a wide range of symptoms and is an unpredictable illness, rheumatologists and lupus experts are invaluable resources. They negotiate the complexities of the illness, modifying plans of care in response to changing symptoms and the patient's reaction to interventions. This flexible approach is essential to maintaining the management strategy's flexibility and responsiveness to the particular difficulties presented by lupus.

To sum up, the foundation of lupus care is made up of rheumatologists and lupus specialists. Their expertise, along with a team-based and patient-focused methodology, establishes a strong foundation for managing the complex aspects of lupus and enhancing patient results.

Assembling Your Medical Staff:

Building a comprehensive healthcare team is essential to navigating the complex world of lupus management. Assembling a team comprising different medical and allied health providers is essential for managing the disease's varied symptoms, in addition to the primary care physician and lupus specialists.

Immunologists are a vital part of this team because they study the complex workings of the immune system and provide insight into the immunological abnormalities that underlie lupus. Their knowledge is crucial for developing therapies that target immune response modulation, which is the mainstay of lupus treatment.

Additionally, considering the frequent cutaneous symptoms linked to lupus, dermatologists should be included. By offering their knowledge in treating cutaneous symptoms, which can range from rashes to more severe manifestations, these specialists help to address the disease's physical and visual components comprehensively.

Working together with nephrologists is essential, particularly when there is significant kidney inflammation, such as lupus nephritis. Their specific expertise guarantees a focused strategy for maintaining renal function, reducing the possible long-term effects on kidney health.

A vital component of the team, psychologists, and counselors understand the emotional toll that long-term conditions like lupus may exact. Their duty involves more than just offering emotional support; it also involves addressing mental health issues, building resilience, and helping with coping mechanisms.

For a comprehensive lupus management strategy to be successful, these varied healthcare providers must work together in concert. A comprehensive and patient-centered approach is fostered by regular communication and coordination, which guarantee that the many aspects of the condition are handled concurrently. Patients' quality of life is improved when their healthcare staff reflects the complex nature of lupus and helps them better negotiate the obstacles the disease presents.

Collaborative Treatment Methods:

A complex and team-based approach to treatment is necessary for the management of lupus, taking into account the complex interactions between symptoms and the individual differences in how each person reacts to therapeutic interventions. This collaborative paradigm entails the patient's educated and active involvement in addition to the active participation of healthcare providers.

Patients and their healthcare team working together to make decisions is one of the main tenets of collaborative treatment. This method makes use of the knowledge of medical specialists while acknowledging the patient's particular experiences and preferences. Patients have a sense of agency and are given the ability to actively participate in decisions that affect their well-being when they are involved in conversations regarding treatment alternatives, possible side effects, and long-term ramifications.

Collaboration also includes coordination and communication between various specialists on the healthcare team, in addition to the interaction between the patient and the healthcare professional. Frequent multidisciplinary conferences provide for a comprehensive comprehension of the patient's state and allow for customized interventions that target the many aspects of lupus. This cooperative synergy makes sure that no facet of the illness is missed, which results in a treatment plan that is more thorough and successful.

When it comes to pharmaceutical interventions, the collaborative approach entails prompt modifications when necessary and close monitoring of the patient's response to medicine. Together, rheumatologists, lupus specialists, and other pertinent medical professionals evaluate how lupus symptoms are changing and adjust medication schedules to minimize adverse effects while controlling symptoms.

Through teamwork, complementary therapies including occupational therapy, physical therapy, and dietary counseling are smoothly included in the treatment plan. These non-pharmacological methods improve general health by addressing the larger effects of lupus on daily living as well as the clinical symptoms.

Essentially, team-based and comprehensive methods of lupus therapy go beyond the conventional patient-physician dynamic. This collaborative mindset acknowledges that the complexity of lupus demands a unified front in which all relevant parties offer their specialized knowledge to attain the best possible results for the patient.

CHAPTER SIX

LUPUS AND MENTAL HEALTH
Understanding the Emotional Impact:

Chronic autoimmune diseases like lupus have a significant effect on a person's mental health in addition to their physical health. Living with lupus has a significant emotional cost since it frequently triggers a wide range of emotions, including dread, worry, despair, and frustration. The unpredictable nature of the illness, with symptoms that might flare up at any time and ongoing anxiety about one's health condition, is one of the main emotional obstacles. People who have lupus may struggle with feeling powerless over their bodies, which can make them feel vulnerable and helpless.

Furthermore, lupus symptoms, both apparent and invisible, can have a big impact on body image and self-esteem. Skin rashes, joint discomfort, and exhaustion can change a person's physical appearance and make it more difficult for them to interact with others, which can exacerbate feelings of loneliness and self-consciousness. Patients may experience increased emotional strain as they go through the complicated maze of treatment plans, prescription drugs, and possible side effects. Because lupus is a chronic condition, people with it must manage their emotions throughout time and reframe their identity to adjust to their "new normal."

Despite these psychological obstacles, raising awareness of the emotional effects of lupus is an essential part of providing comprehensive care. It makes it possible for patients, their families, and medical experts to identify and deal with the psychological effects of the illness.

Support networks, educational materials, and honest discussions about mental health issues can help create a more knowledgeable and compassionate community that recognizes and validates the emotional challenges brought on by lupus.

Adaptive coping mechanisms are essential for navigating the psychological and physical obstacles that lupus presents. Coping strategies are essential for enhancing the quality of life for people with lupus because they enable them to overcome hardship with fortitude and resiliency. First and foremost, one of the most important coping strategies is knowledge of the illness and how to treat it. Being aware of the symptoms, causes, and available treatments enables people to take an active role in their care, which promotes empowerment and a sense of control.

Maintaining a healthy lifestyle also becomes essential for managing lupus. Healthy eating, getting enough sleep, and exercising regularly all improve general well-being and reduce certain symptoms. Stress-reduction methods like yoga, meditation, and mindfulness are vital components of the coping strategies for lupus patients. Since stress has been linked to lupus flare-ups, managing stress is essential for controlling symptoms.

Creating a solid support network is another essential coping strategy. Making connections with people who are aware of the difficulties associated with having lupus, whether via online forums or support groups, makes one feel less alone and gives one a sense of community. Friends and family can provide social support that helps people deal with the ups and downs of living with lupus and promotes emotional well-being.

Effective coping strategies for lupus are ultimately individualized and may include a mix of self-care routines, emotional support, and lifestyle modifications. By incorporating these techniques into daily life, people can take charge of their health and improve their quality of life in general.

Looking for Expert Assistance:

Obtaining expert assistance is an essential part of receiving comprehensive care in the complicated world of lupus. While treating the physical symptoms of lupus typically receives the majority of medical attention, treating the mental health component calls for specific training. Psychologists, psychiatrists, and counselors are examples of mental health experts who can provide helpful assistance in overcoming the emotional difficulties brought on by lupus.

Examining and treating the psychological effects of a chronic illness is one important advantage of getting expert help. Experts can assist people in managing their feelings, creating coping mechanisms, and strengthening their ability to bounce back from setbacks. In particular, cognitive-behavioral therapy has demonstrated the potential to support people with chronic illnesses by reframing their negative thought patterns and assisting them in creating useful coping skills.

Furthermore, family members and caregivers are included in the professional support system in addition to the individual. Relationships are frequently strained by lupus, so enrolling loved ones in therapy or counseling can improve understanding and communication. As duties and responsibilities change to fit the difficulties of living with lupus, family dynamics may change as well. Expert counsel can help with this adjustment process.

Psychiatrists may be quite helpful in diagnosing and prescribing the right medications when it comes to managing mental health issues with medication. A holistic approach to health is promoted by incorporating mental health services into the entire lupus treatment plan, which recognizes the connection between physical and emotional well-being.

In general, getting help from a specialist for mental health and lupus is a proactive step in receiving complete care. It acknowledges the complex nature of the illness and places a high value on people's mental health and the health of their support systems, building resilience and encouraging a better quality of life despite the difficulties that lupus presents.

CHAPTER SEVEN

LUPUS AND NUTRITION
Anti-Inflammatory Food Plan:

Developing an anti-inflammatory diet is essential to effectively control the symptoms of lupus. Inflammation is a hallmark of lupus, an autoimmune disease, and various foods can either reduce or increase inflammatory reactions. Eating foods with anti-inflammatory qualities is the main goal of an anti-inflammatory diet, which also attempts to lessen the effects of lupus on different organs by decreasing inflammation in the body.

Include fruits and vegetables high in antioxidants, such as tomatoes, leafy greens, and berries, in an anti-inflammatory diet for lupus patients. These foods aid in the elimination of free radicals, which may be a factor in inflammation. Furthermore, it has been demonstrated that omega-3 fatty acids, which are present in flaxseeds and fatty fish like salmon, have anti-inflammatory properties that may help people with lupus.

On the other hand, pro-inflammatory foods including processed meals, red meat, and large amounts of refined carbohydrates should be avoided by lupus sufferers. These foods may exacerbate lupus symptoms by causing inflammation. By following a varied and well-balanced diet and avoiding certain triggers, people with lupus can take control of their health and lessen the frequency and intensity of flare-ups.

Another tactic to increase the anti-inflammatory potential of a lupus-friendly diet is to include anti-inflammatory herbs and spices like ginger and turmeric in meals. These components have anti-inflammatory qualities due to their bioactive molecules, which improve the general health of lupus patients.

In essence, choosing a nutrient-dense, anti-inflammatory diet for lupus entails minimizing the consumption of pro-inflammatory foods and making thoughtful, deliberate food selections. For people with lupus, this dietary strategy is essential for controlling inflammation, reducing symptoms, and enhancing overall quality of life.

Supplements for the Treatment of Lupus:

Supplements are a valuable tool in the overall management of lupus, as they offer vital nutrients that may be lacking in the diet or difficult to obtain on their own. While it's important for lupus sufferers to speak with their doctors before starting any new supplement regimen, several supplements have demonstrated potential in helping manage lupus and reducing particular symptoms.

Vitamin D is an essential supplement for people with lupus. Vitamin D deficiency is common in lupus patients, and supplementation can help resolve this issue. Maintaining sufficient levels of vitamin D can help lower the risk of osteoporosis, which is a worry for some lupus patients, particularly those on long-term corticosteroid therapy. Vitamin D is needed for bone health.

Fish oil capsules and other omega-3 fatty acid supplements contain anti-inflammatory qualities that may help reduce lupus-related inflammation. Supplementing with these can help increase the amount of foods high in omega-3 fatty acids in your diet.

Furthermore, certain antioxidants like vitamins C and E may help minimize inflammation and counteract oxidative stress in people with lupus. But it's important to find a balance because taking too many supplements might have negative effects.

Probiotics are another type of probiotic that may be helpful for people with lupus since they promote intestinal health. An increasing corpus of evidence points to a link between autoimmune illnesses and the gut microbiome and implies that keeping the gut flora in a healthy balance may have immune-boosting effects.

In summary, supplements can be useful additions to a lupus treatment plan, but their use needs to be customized to each patient's needs and closely monitored under the supervision of medical specialists. A comprehensive approach to managing this intricate autoimmune disease includes a well-informed approach to supplementation, along with other components of lupus care and a balanced diet.

Dietary Influence on Symptoms:

The intricate connection between nutrition and lupus symptoms has important consequences for people living with this inflammatory disease. An intelligent and customized diet can affect energy levels, affect the frequency and intensity of lupus flares, and improve general health.

Dietary factors primarily impact lupus symptoms by modulating inflammation. It has been demonstrated that some meals, especially those high in omega-3 fatty acids and antioxidants, have anti-inflammatory qualities. People with lupus may see a decrease in inflammation by including these items in their diet, which could result in a decrease in the frequency and severity of their symptoms.

On the other hand, meals that promote inflammation, such as those heavy in sugar and saturated fats, can worsen inflammation and cause lupus flare-ups. For lupus patients, avoiding or reducing certain foods is an essential part of diet management. It's also critical to maintain a healthy weight with a balanced diet since being overweight can exacerbate lupus symptoms like fatigue and joint discomfort.

Beyond inflammation, many lupus symptoms including skin rashes and photosensitivity can be influenced by food. Certain meals, such as those strong in histamines or chemicals, can exacerbate skin-related symptoms for some lupus patients. People with lupus can better control and alleviate these particular signs by recognizing and avoiding trigger foods.

A nutrient-rich diet is even more important when taking into account the possible adverse effects of pharmaceuticals like corticosteroids, which are frequently prescribed for lupus. People with lupus must concentrate on foods that support bone health and fill in any nutritional gaps because some drugs have the potential to cause bone loss or nutritional deficits.

To sum up, there are several ways that food affects lupus symptoms, including controlling inflammation, controlling weight, and addressing particular triggers. With the help of a tailored strategy directed by medical experts and based on individual feedback, people with lupus can use diet to improve their general health and quality of life.

CHAPTER EIGHT

LUPUS WARRIORS: ADAPTING THEIR LIFESTYLES
Managing Exercise and Rest:

A crucial lifestyle modification for people with lupus is striking a careful balance between exercise and rest. An autoimmune condition called lupus frequently causes symptoms like weakening in the muscles, joint discomfort, and exhaustion. Maintaining this chronic disease requires finding the ideal mix between being active and providing enough rest.

Lupus warriors must pay attention to their bodies and identify symptoms of exhaustion or elevated discomfort. Walking, swimming, or yoga are examples of moderate, low-impact workouts that can help maintain muscular strength and joint flexibility without being too strenuous. Realizing one's limitations is also important, though. The symptoms of lupus can be made worse by overexertion, which can result in flare-ups and increased inflammation. Therefore, it's crucial to pace activities and include rest periods.

Additionally, sleep is essential for controlling lupus symptoms. Having a regular sleep schedule and getting enough restorative sleep can have a good effect on general well-being. Making good sleep a priority can help reduce fatigue, which is a typical lupus symptom. Improved sleep hygiene can be attained by making a sleep-friendly environment, practicing relaxation techniques before bed, and abstaining from stimulants.

Lupus warriors need to adopt an adaptable mindset to successfully navigate the complex dance between exertion and rest. Being flexible is essential since symptoms might change and daily schedules must be modified. Personalized activity programs that are in line with each person's goals and health circumstances can be developed with the help of medical professionals like physical therapists and rheumatologists. Essentially, finding the right balance between exercise and relaxation is a dynamic process that is customized to meet the individual needs of every lupus warrior rather than a one-size-fits-all strategy.

Handling Tension:

One of the most important lifestyle changes for people with lupus is stress management. Both physical and mental stress have been linked to an increased risk of lupus flare-ups and exacerbation of pre-existing symptoms. As such, implementing stress-reduction strategies that work is essential to improving general well-being.

Deep breathing exercises and other mindfulness and relaxation practices can be effective strategies for reducing stress. These techniques have a beneficial effect on the body's physiological reaction to stress by easing emotional tension and fostering a sense of calm. Yoga and tai chi, for example, which combine mindfulness and physical exercise, can also be effective holistic methods of stress relief for lupus sufferers.

Two essential elements of stress management are reasonable expectations and effective communication. Warriors with lupus may encounter difficulties performing everyday tasks that others might take for granted. Fostering understanding and support can be achieved by keeping lines of communication open with friends, family, and employers. Preventing unneeded pressures requires admitting one's limitations and setting realistic objectives and goals.

The emotional toll of having a chronic illness can be explored and managed by lupus warriors in a secure environment with the help of professional care, such as counseling or therapy. Including stress-relieving activities in everyday routines, like taking up a hobby, going on a nature walk, or spending time with loved ones, helps build resilience overall against the difficulties that come with having lupus.

Creating a Helpful Network:

For those with lupus, creating a strong and encouraging network is essential to managing and overcoming the obstacles this autoimmune condition presents. The battle with lupus is not just physical but also emotional and psychological, and having a strong support network can greatly enhance one's quality of life in general.

Friends and family are essential sources of understanding and emotional support. Teaching others in intimate circles about lupus, its symptoms, and possible obstacles promotes empathy and establishes a supportive environment for lupus warriors. Setting clear expectations and boundaries for each person requires open and honest communication.

Joining lupus communities or support groups can provide a feeling of shared experience and belonging in addition to personal interactions. These platforms offer a forum for exchanging perspectives, coping mechanisms, and emotional support with people who understand the day-to-day complexities of living with lupus. This extended network can be built with the help of national organizations that advocate for lupus, local support groups, and online forums.

Healthcare experts, such as rheumatologists, nurses, and mental health specialists, constitute an additional vital layer of assistance. Effective communication and frequent check-ins with the medical team guarantee that lupus warriors receive thorough treatment and are given the tools they need to effectively manage their health.

It is essential to give lupus patients the tools they need to actively seek out and maintain their support system. A strong support system can be an effective tool in the fight against lupus by fostering empathy, sharing experiences, and educating others. It can also lead to better mental and physical health as well as an overall higher standard of living.

CHAPTER NINE

LUPUS AND PREGNANCY
Getting Ready for a Baby:

Pregnancy planning is an essential step for women with lupus since it necessitates thoughtful planning and proactive management to guarantee a favorable outcome for the mother and the unborn child. Due to the autoimmune nature of lupus, which can affect fertility and raise the risk of problems, women who have the disease frequently encounter particular difficulties during conception and pregnancy.

First and foremost, before trying to become pregnant, women with lupus must speak with their medical staff. Rheumatologists, obstetricians, and other experts who can offer thorough advice specific to the patient's health situation usually make up this team. Developing a customized plan that reduces risks during pregnancy requires evaluating the woman's overall health, her lupus activity, and her existing medications.

Medication adjustments are an important factor to take into account when planning. It might be necessary to modify or replace certain widely prescribed drugs for lupus symptoms with safer options to protect the developing fetus and the mother. A fine balance must be struck between limiting the baby's risk of injury and managing lupus activity.

Throughout the planning phase, careful observation and frequent evaluations are necessary. This entails monitoring lupus activity, swiftly managing any possible flare-ups, and making sure the woman's general health continues to be at its best. Preconception counseling can also offer helpful advice on lifestyle elements that can lead to a better pregnancy, like stress management and nutrition.

It is essential to inform the woman and others close to her about the possible obstacles and precautions to take. Preventive actions can be made to ensure a safer and more successful pregnancy by realizing the significance of early prenatal care, leading a healthy lifestyle, and identifying warning signs.

In conclusion, a woman with lupus must work in tandem with her medical team and support system when preparing for pregnancy. Optimal odds of a safe pregnancy and birth can be achieved with a complete strategy that includes open communication, careful monitoring, and medication modifications.

Pregnancy Hazards And Their Handling:

Due to the autoimmune nature of lupus, pregnant women with the disease face particular difficulties. To maximize difficulties and ensure a successful pregnancy, it is imperative to recognize and manage the potential hazards.

The possibility of flare-ups or worsening of lupus symptoms is one of the main worries for women with lupus during pregnancy. Pregnancy may cause modifications to the immune system, which is already hyperactive in lupus patients, which could exacerbate the condition. Consequently, it is essential to closely monitor lupus activity through routine check-ups and consultations with medical professionals.

Furthermore, women with lupus have an increased chance of developing preeclampsia, premature birth, and fetal development limitation, among other pregnancy concerns. This highlights how crucial it is to receive specialist prenatal care and regular monitoring to identify and quickly address any possible problems. Reducing these risks may require changing lifestyle choices, taking different medications, and working closely with obstetricians and rheumatologists.

It is a hard effort to manage lupus symptoms while also considering the needs of the developing fetus. Pregnant women should carefully assess the risks associated with certain regularly used lupus drugs and, in some situations, make necessary changes. To identify a drug regimen that minimizes potential risk to the unborn child while effectively controlling lupus activity, close collaboration with healthcare experts is essential.

One of the most important aspects of managing a lupus pregnancy is teaching the expectant mother about self-care and warning flags. A proactive approach to ensuring a safer pregnancy includes stressing the value of following doctor's orders, leading a healthy lifestyle, and getting help right away if something seems off.

To summarize, the management of pregnancy risks in lupus-affected women entails close observation, teamwork in the medical setting, and an individualized approach to medication and lifestyle modifications. Many lupus-afflicted women can conceive successfully and give birth to healthy children with the right care.

For lupus-affected women, the postpartum phase necessitates close monitoring and continued medical assistance to manage the particular difficulties and possible consequences that may develop following childbirth. Postpartum concerns are not limited to the delivery process; they center on the health of the mother and the infant.

Keeping an eye out for possible flare-ups of lupus is a crucial part of postpartum care for women with lupus. After childbirth, there can be hormonal swings and immune system modifications that can set off lupus symptoms. To quickly detect and handle any new symptoms or concerns, women during the postpartum period must maintain continuous communication with their healthcare providers.

In the postpartum period, ongoing cooperation between obstetricians and rheumatologists is crucial. Depending on the mother's health and whether she is nursing, the medication regimen may need to be modified. The safety of nursing must be balanced with the requirement for continued lupus control, which calls for serious thought and candid consultation with medical specialists.

Many new mothers worry about postpartum depression, and women with lupus may be more susceptible. Feelings of being overwhelmed can be exacerbated by the mental and physical strain of managing a chronic condition in addition to the responsibilities of caring for a newborn. Consequently, to quickly diagnose and treat postpartum depression, mental health assistance and routine check-ins with healthcare professionals are essential.

For women with lupus, breastfeeding issues are important in postpartum care. Even though breastfeeding is often advised due to its many health advantages, some drugs used to treat lupus symptoms may find their way into breast milk. The advantages and disadvantages of breastfeeding can be carefully considered in consultation with medical professionals, enabling an informed choice that puts the health of the mother and the welfare of the child first.

To sum up, postpartum care for lupus-affected women includes careful breastfeeding decision-making, continued medical monitoring, and mental health support. Women with lupus can successfully manage the difficulties of the postpartum phase and have a happy, healthy experience as new mothers if they receive thorough postpartum care.

CHAPTER TEN

STUDIES AND PROSPECTS
Current Studies on Lupus:

Recent years have seen tremendous progress in the field of lupus research toward solving the intricate riddles underlying this autoimmune condition. Understanding the underlying causes, hereditary variables, and molecular processes involved in the pathogenesis of lupus has been the focus of research. Finding certain biomarkers that may help with early diagnosis and illness progression prediction is one important field of research. This allows for timely intervention, which could transform the management of lupus.

Moreover, new directions for targeted therapeutics have been made possible by developments in immunology and molecular biology. The goal now is to reduce the side effects of traditional immunosuppressive treatments by creating medications that specifically alter the immune response. Novel approaches, such as CRISPR gene editing, are being investigated to rectify lupus-related genetic defects, perhaps leading to more individualized and efficient therapies.

Comprehensive lupus databases have been established as a result of cooperative efforts within the world's scientific community, which has encouraged data exchange and expanded our understanding of the illness. This collaborative method facilitates the detection of similarities and variances in lupus symptoms among varied groups, while also speeding up research.

As we commemorate the first anniversary of our ongoing pursuit of knowledge, it is imperative to recognize the collaborative efforts that have catapulted lupus research into an unprecedented realm of opportunities. In addition to providing the groundwork for revolutionary discoveries, these endeavors give hope to the millions of people afflicted with lupus worldwide.

Innovative therapeutic techniques that have the potential to improve patient outcomes are changing the face of lupus treatment. One important discovery is the creation of targeted biologics, which target particular immune system components implicated in the pathophysiology of lupus. By reducing the side effects of conventional immunosuppressive drugs, these biologics seek to offer more targeted and effective therapies.

Small-molecule inhibitors are being investigated as a potential therapy option for lupus in addition to biologics. By focusing on important signaling channels connected to the immune response, these substances provide a more sophisticated and individualized method of treating the illness. Clinical trials are being conducted to evaluate the safety and effectiveness of these innovative treatments, offering a ray of hope to those facing the difficulties associated with lupus.

Additionally, developments in stem cell therapy and regenerative medicine are being studied as possible game-changers in the treatment of lupus. Regenerative medicine presents a promising new way to manage lupus and enhance patient quality of life by regenerating damaged tissues and adjusting the immune system.

Looking back over the last year, it's clear that the treatment landscape for lupus is about to undergo a radical shift. Researchers, doctors, and pharmaceutical companies are working tirelessly to advance the area so that successful, targeted lupus medicines become a reality in the future.

Promoting Awareness of Lupus and Advocacy:

In the larger lupus community, advocacy is essential because it acts as a spark for better patient care, more funding for research, and raised awareness. There has been a determined attempt in the last year to raise the voices of lupus patients in the public and the community.

Campaigns have aimed to de-stigmatize the condition, debunk misconceptions, and create a community that supports people dealing with lupus.

In the field of policymaking, activists have dedicated their lives to obtaining more money for lupus research and making sure that the needs of lupus sufferers are given top priority in healthcare legislation. This entails promoting better access to specialized treatment, reasonably priced drugs, and a deeper comprehension of the particular difficulties experienced by lupus sufferers.

Digital platforms such as social media have shown to be effective instruments for increasing awareness of lupus. Online activism has been essential in reaching a larger audience and building a feeling of community, ranging from personal tales published by people living with lupus to educational efforts highlighting the realities of the condition.

It is clear that progress has been achieved as we approach the one-year mark of our lobbying activities, but more work has to be done.

There is a resolute dedication to lupus advocacy, with a shared goal to keep promoting improvements, dismantling obstacles, and making sure that lupus gets the resources and attention it requires on a worldwide basis.

www.ingramcontent.com/pod-product-compliance
Lightning Source LLC
Chambersburg PA
CBHW050745260726
48661CB00001B/430